The Lost Book of Herbal Remedies

Rediscovering Nature's Healing Powers

LI MINGHAO

Table of Contents

Table of Contents 5

Foreword 9

The Roots of Healing 13

The Dawn of Herbal Medicine 14

Nature's Pharmacy: A Global Tapestry 15

The Wisdom of Ancestors 16

The Evolution of Herbal Remedies through the Ages 17

The Herbal Pantheon 21

Profiles of Power: A Selection of Key Herbs 22

The Science of Plant Medicine 31

Unveiling Phytochemistry: The Compounds Behind the Cure 31

Herbal Synergy: The Entourage Effect in Plant Medicine 33

From Plant to Prescription: The Journey of Herbal Compounds 35

Clinical Trials and Herbal Efficacy 36

Cultivating Your Herbal Garden 39

Getting Started: Planning Your Herbal Garden 40

Choosing Herbs Based on Therapeutic Needs and Organic Gardening Practices 42

Pest Control: Natural Solutions for a Healthy Garden 43

The Timing of Harvesting Your Herbs and Methods of Preservation 44

Harvesting and Storing Your Bounty 47

The Art of Timing: When to Harvest Your Herbs — 48

Harvesting Techniques: Doing It Right — 48

Post-Harvest Handling, Drying, and Storage — 50

Organising Your Home Apothecary Stock — 51

Herbal Remedies for Everyday Ailments 53

Nature's Medicine Cabinet: An Overview — 54

The Art of Herbal Preparation 61

Mastering Herbal Concoctions and Infusions — 62

Medicinal Uses of Herbal Extracts, Infusions, and Tinctures — 64

Making Herbal Capsules and Powders — 65

Making Herbal Syrups and Elixirs — 66

Herbal Recipes and Formulations...............69

Specialized Formulations for Immune Support — 70

Formulations for Anxiety Relief That Induce Sleep — 73

Making a Poultice — 74

Herbalism in Daily Life 77

Everyday Herbalism: Making It a Lifestyle — 77

Herbs in Nutrition and Cooking — 79

Nighttime Rituals With Herbs — 81

Teaching Herbalism to Family and Friends — 82

Mind, Body, and Spirit 85

The Holistic Philosophy of Herbalism — 85

Spiritual and Meditative Uses of Herbs — 87

The Ethics of Herbalism 93

Understanding Ethical Herbalism — 94

Wildcrafting and Other Sustainable Sourcing practices   95

Cultural Respect and Avoiding Appropriation   98

The Global Herbal Movement 99

Herbalism in the Modern World   99

Bridging Tradition and Innovation   100

Cross-Cultural Exchange of Herbal Knowledge   101

Advocacy and Community in Herbalism   104

Building Your Herbal Community 107

The Importance of Community in Herbalism   107

Participation in Sharing Circles and Study Groups   109

Engaging With Professional Herbalists and Leaders   111

The Herbalist's Toolkit.............................113

Essential Tools for the Herbalist   113

Building Your Herbal Reference Library With Digital Resources   115

Tracking Your Herbal Journey   116

Conclusion   117

Glossary 121

References 125

Foreword

Ever wondered why humanity has drifted away from its wealth of traditional knowledge amid rising dependence on modern medicine? Well, the advancements of the twentieth century made life easier for us, but tied our fate with the use of drugs to stay healthy. There is more to modern medicine than meets the eye, as the side effects of these drugs and the reliance on processed foods have contributed to the rise of rare diseases, such as celiac disease, and autoimmune disorders that were not present in the human population till the twentieth century. The incidence of autism spectrum disorders, autoimmune disorders, and rare diseases has substantially increased since the past 50 years. This has been further aggravated by the overabundance of plastics and chemicals that we inadvertently ingest everyday. Teflon, which is chemically polytetrafluoroethylene, is used to coat frying pans and pots to provide a non-stick surface. Owned by Chemours, a spinoff from DuPont Chemical Company, teflon gets scraped off as by the use of the spatula as you cook and becomes a part of the food we eat. The solution to this problem is simple: we need to return to the ways of our ancestors that relied on nature to do everything. The overuse of modern advancements have made us susceptible to a range of problems, so we need to turn back to mother nature. This book splays out the solutions that you can incorporate in your life to rid yourself of the downside of the modern world.

Herbalism and ancient traditional knowledge can be used in conjunction with modern medicine in an effort to attain the goals of holistic health, which targets the mind, body, and spirit as a single, interconnected entity. Traditional Chinese medicine serves as the beating heart of this book and it is widely practiced to this day. Ethical and sustainable cultivation practices are encouraged throughout the subject-matter of this book, so much so that wildcrafting can also be considered an option when you run out of ingredients at your home. The scope of this book restricts the use of chemicals in our ultra-commodified world. Health-conscious individuals and enthusiasts of herbal remedies will find that these practices resonate with their heart. This book guides you to the ways you can ethically and sustainably grow medicinally important herbs. Involvement in communities and online spaces lends you a feeling of belonging, as you communicate with a galore of like-minded people that make it easy for you keep abreast with the latest trends in the realm of herbalism. The art of making poultices, potions, salves, and infusions has been detailed in this book along with ways you can harvest your herbal bounty in copious amounts. Keeping your plants in viable shape post-harvest is highly imperative for another successful growing season, which is especially true for perennial plants. Tried and tested methods that can make your garden abound with herbs have been etched onto the pages of this book. Keeping a stack of books on herbal knowledge can serve as an indispensable scaffold for your knowledge to reach new heights, and relevant journal articles about research in this field can further amplify your understanding of herbal medicine.

Still vacillating between the decision of purchasing or leaving this book on the shelf? This book is full of gems that have been interspersed throughout its pages using the knowledge of Li Minghao.

Li Minghao hails from Yunnan, China. This is a region known for its rich herbal heritage and biodiversity. His upbringing in this environment oozing with traditional herbal knowledge predisposed him to learn a lot about the use of herbs to alleviate common ailments. His affection for traditional medicine reflects from the fact that he pursued formal education in botany and Chinese medicine. His travels took him across the two continents, where he learned about different cultural influences on traditional knowledge. He is dedicated to a harmonious connection with nature that promotes holistic well-being.

So, dive deep into the depths of this book to discover the gems that can alter your way of thinking and take you to a land that has become lost to mankind!

Chapter 1
The Roots of Healing

Though modern medicine was steered into existence almost a century ago by Andrew Carnegie and a handful of other philanthropists and industrialists, herbal medicine has been the bedrock of civilisation since antiquity. Plants have had a major role in the treatment of disease throughout the ages, and numerous systems of medicine pertinent to different cultures sprouted into existence. The underlying philosophical premise might be dissimilar for these systems of medicine; however, the undeniable role that herbs have played in the treatment of disease cannot be overlooked. Egypt, Mesopotamia, and the Orient (China, Japan, and Tibet) have been the epicentres of the growth of civilisations, and developed unique systems of medicine with varying philosophical cornerstone. The Unani (طب یونانی - Islamic) and Ayurvedic (Hindu) systems of medicine have also played a role in shaping modern Western medicine. Therefore, the botanical and pharmacognostics evaluation of these medicinal plants is important to comprehend their healing properties. This stretch of this book immerses you in the rich history of herbalism, which is critical to the way you would evaluate the use of herbs to treat common ailments.

The Dawn of Herbal Medicine

Cultures and religions have shown stark contrast in the way they processed herbal and medicinal information, and this was primarily due to the differences in revered philosophical thought related to the region. It was a commonplace occurrence for a particular person to display resounding intellect and specialise in numerous fields of philosophy. This is how the term polymath was coined, as this term refers to an intellectual who possesses a great depth of knowledge about different branches of philosophical thought. For instance, Avicenna is a revered Muslim polymath of his time who published his magnum opus, *Kitab-al-Shifa*, wherein he documented the curative properties of medicinal plants and their use in different diseases. Luckily, his work survived the Mongol invasion and destruction of Baghdad led by Ogedei Khan. The use of parchment was the principal form of materialising information, as printing presses were plunged into existence only 400 years later, c. 1440 AD. The Golden Age of Islam gave birth to, and significantly developed, medicine as a field. Later on, Europe and Caucasian influence intervened after emerging from the Dark Ages, and considerably transformed medicine into a complex entity that we witness today.

The only system of herbal medicine that truly persisted and flourished throughout the advancement of modern medicine is the Chinese system of herbal medicine. A substantial number of people still practice this form of medicine in China, and other ethnic groups, such as the Indochinese of South East Asia, also revere this system of medicine. There has been significant controversy around the use of Chinese medicine, but that did not thwart people from using it to cure illnesses. Poaching used to be an illegal activity that was hard to police, but trophy hunting of aged lions has diluted the controversial use of lion bones in Chinese medicine, as trophy hunting significantly drives the conservation efforts centred around the species as a whole. Also, hunters get to sell the lion bones at exorbitant rates in China, creating a non-zero-sum game for all parties involved in this scenario. Illegal poaching activities are now dwindling in numbers, and therefore, do not let this factor dissuade you from your desire to indulge in Chinese herbal medicine.

Nature's Pharmacy: A Global Tapestry

The natural world has purveyed mankind an incessant supply of herbal plants. This can be likened to the coloured threads of a tapestry that are interwoven to create an image that represents the harmonious connection between nature and mankind. Utilisation of the phytochemical compounds present in the herbs not only mitigates and cures diseases, but also augments the normal physiological function of the body, so much so that your body feels rejuvenated and enlivened.

Much consideration has been given to the extraction of these phytochemicals from new species of plants and their extensive study in order to splay out and probe the organ system effects that are induced in humans. The chemical structures of the well-known compounds have been determined, thereby making synthetic production of these compounds very easy.

The Wisdom of Ancestors

The use of parchment and clay tablets has been crucial to transmit herbal knowledge and wisdom of ancestors throughout history. The first British Pharmacopeia was printed in 1864 in London, which standardised herbal knowledge through the use of specific dose regimens and routes of administration for the drugs. However, this was only possible because herbal knowledge had already undergone significant scrutiny through the Middle Ages and the Renaissance. The Renaissance oversaw a period of substantial growth in the knowledge of mankind. Many new scientists hailing from that chronological period made their name through significant ground-breaking discoveries about the human body. The exploration of the biological and chemical realm inspired the creation of fictional characters, such as Sherlock Holmes. Robert Hooke made the serendipitous discovery of cells when he observed a piece of cork under the microscope. Since printing presses had already been established in that time, the new discoveries of that time were much easy to document by these scientists.

The Evolution of Herbal Remedies through the Ages

There has been a resurgence of interest in herbal remedies in the contemporary society. Cosmetic chemists and pharmacists now seek to include natural ingredients in cosmetics. The consumers have also gravitated toward the use of products that include natural herbal ingredients. Kiehl's is one of the foremost cosmetic companies that incorporates naturally-derived ingredients in their products. Their anti-aging cream makes use of chaga mushroom that boosts radiance and refines skin tone. Avon, L'Oréal, Lancôme, Clinique and other huge names use herbal extracts in their products.

The fact that herbal compounds have been key to the development of modern medicine has been disseminated through throughout the twentieth century, thereby making the use of herbal extracts and their synthetic derivatives acceptable for the general public. The scientific validation of these remedies has been made available to the public ever since the culmination of the Second World War.

Although natural herbs are no longer being used in medicines and cosmetics, they play a crucial role in modern healthcare technology. Herbs were used to characterise the medicinal phytochemicals that are found in them and to further study the way that these compounds trigger the cell-signalling pathways and physiologic mechanisms in the human body. Therefore, herbs remain indispensable repository of a colossal data set that remains to be explored even further. There are huge swathes of uncharted territories within the herbs and plants that have not been studied, and there is a galore of plants that still remains unknown to the botanical system that has been devised by humans.

Drug discovery studies are carried out for research and development of new molecules that can cure diseases that do not have any cure to this day, and to enhance the life expectancy of patients where palliative treatments are the main focus of the therapeutic regimen. Actual herbs are no longer used for the extraction of these phytochemicals, as these compounds are found in very meager amounts, and using the herbs for the extraction of compounds becomes a very expensive process. As the structural morphology of the useful medicinal phytochemicals has already been debunked, these compounds are produced by organic synthesis. This is a man-made chemical process that is carried out on a large-scale in the research labs of biotechnology and pharmaceutical companies.

Indubitably, herbs have always been the main source for extraction and study of useful compounds that can improve the quality of life. There are many regions in the world that resort to the use of raw herbs to alleviate ailments. Potions are made from the herbal plants that are applied topically on the wound or site of infection. This is why herbal remedies are now being brought back to life in the West as well, as these remedies can be very effective for alleviating common ailments.

Chapter 2
The Herbal Pantheon

Although there is a litany of herbs that have been identified through binomial nomenclature, a few herbs stand out as being the most important among their counterparts. This is because some herbs are rich in many phytochemicals that have been very well-researched and known to cure, or have mitigating effects on, numerous illnesses. Such herbs can be taken for a variety of ailments to produce the desired alleviating effect. These herbs have been revered by our ancestors since ancient times. Although these herbs are known to have an effect on a number of illnesses, some people have resorted to creating myths about their healing properties that have served to do nothing except add to the reverence of these plants. Some ancient traditions live on to this day and can be seen among some cultures across the globe. One important thing to note is that seasonal variations can alter the concentrations of the phytochemicals in all herbs, so careful attention must be given to this characteristic of the herbs, as you need to be able to have a herb rich in the sought-after phytochemical for optimum effect.

Profiles of Power: A Selection of Key Herbs

There is a cornucopia of herbs that have proven health benefits, but you need to focus on only those herbs that can be easily and sustainably grown in your backyard. Also, you need to use these herbs only for adults, as the organ system effects induced by these herbs can vary in children and pregnant women. The World Health Organization has a List of Basic and Essential Drugs that is comprised of 11% drugs that are purely of plant origin. The fact that all of the other drugs have been synthesised keeping the effects of the naturally found drugs in mind is key for you to be used as a motivation to delve deep into the world of herbal medicine. Some key herbs have been detailed in this chapter.

Gingko

Gingko is one of the oldest herbs that have been known to man. it has considerable importance in Chinese medicine. Phenols and phenolic glycosides are found in many herbal plants, and although the detailed constituents of gingko have not been known, it is believed that it is rich in these compounds. This is because anthocyanins, flavonoids and flavones are classified as anthraquinones, and gingko has been found to be rich in flavonoids. Flavonoids can be present as pharmacologically inactive constituents, but many flavonoid-containing herbs have

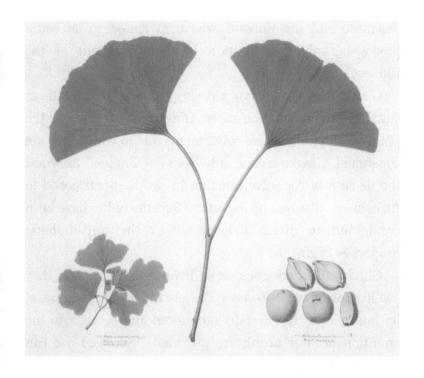

them as active constituents. Many flavonoid-rich herbs have been included in the British Pharmacopeia as well. Many others have already been on the British Herbal Compendium, BHP.

This tree is indigenous to China, but has been extensively traded along the Silk Route for centuries, and can now be found everywhere on the planet. It is planted along the roadside, as its fan-shaped leaves add to the scenic beauty of the region. The tree started to be cultivated by the Chinese almost a thousands years ago, particularly due to its rare occurrence. It first grabbed the attention of the

Japanese and the Koreans who contributed to its wider phylogeographic distribution by following suit of the Chinese.

Gingko leaves undergo a drying process to make them suitable for consumption as tea. Gingko nuts contain all the pharmacologically active constituents due to which they are consumed. Gingko has already been documented to retard the decline in cognitive function in people predisposed to Alzheimer's disease and dementia. Recent studies have been conducted to discover more about the anti-diabetic properties of gingko.

Gingko tress are considered living fossils because they can live for up to 3000 years. Despite the benefits of gingko, its intake must be carefully monitored and brought to the attention of your healthcare provider. Prolonged use can alter the function of liver microsomal cytochrome P450s, which are enzymes that are critical to the processes of metabolism and biotransformation of drugs. Liver cancer can also develop due to prolonged use. Also, gingko seeds are poisonous and must be disposed of carefully if you decide to grow gingko in your backyard.

Turmeric

Turmeric has been used as a condiment for centuries by mankind. Turmeric is indigenous to the Indian subcontinent and contains many useful compounds that have anti-tumor properties that thwart the progression of cancers. The compounds that it contains prevent mutations in the DNA.

The delicious taste that turmeric lends to many dishes makes it a very famous condiment, and is used in marinades as well. It has many anti-inflammatory compounds that make it useful for patients of osteoarthritis. One important thing to consider is that turmeric has considerably low bioavailability, and therefore, it is consumed with pepper to enhance the absorption of its constituents.

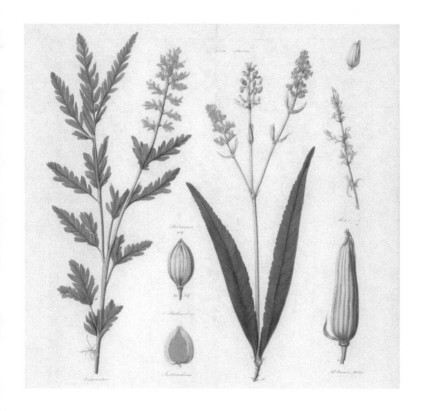

Evening Primrose Oil

Evening primrose oil has a cornucopia of benefits that are not just limited to the consumption of the oil. It is also used for cooking oil and offers an upper hand over canola and sunflower oil owing to its high smoking point. Smoking point is related to the number of free fatty acids found in the oil. As oils heat up, the free fatty acids are released, which are then broken down to produce smoke as the temperature gets higher. The acid value of an oil is the grams of potassium hydroxide required to neutralise the free fatty

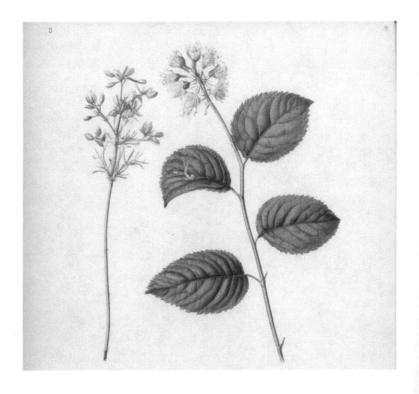

acids, and a low acid value oil is also used in parenteral dosage forms of drugs (injections). A high smoking point value for an oil simply means that food can be cooked quickly at higher temperatures.

Evening primrose oil can alleviate the symptoms of premenstrual syndrome (PMS) and polycystic ovary syndrome (PCOS) in women. The pain associated with tender breasts can also be mitigated. Other than that, applying the oil topically on the skin can alleviate the symptoms of various skin conditions, such as atopic dermatitis and eczema.

Professional consultation of qualified healthcare providers must be sough before taking this oil in any form, as it can alter drug absorption for patients of AIDS, and can also alter the absorption of lithium in patients of bipolar disorder.

Flaxseed

Flaxseeds are very commonly ingested by people owing to their antioxidant and anti-inflammatory effects. These seeds are also added to muesli and oatmeal bowls to make the meal more healthy. They are also attributed to the reduction of obesity.

Recent clinical research has been focused on the effect of flaxseeds in cancers, and it has been found that they reduce the progression of colon cancer. Flaxseeds are consumed in various ways other than the ones discussed above, as they

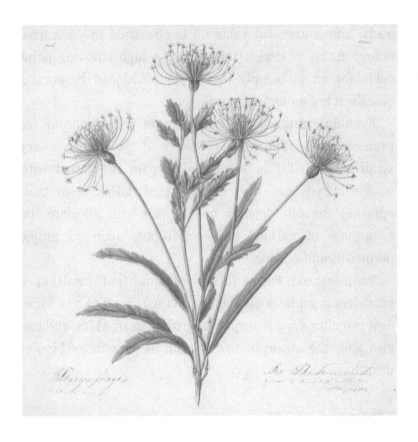

can be added yogurt, salad dressings, and also eaten just as they are without adding them to anything.

Tea Tree Oil

Tea tree is indigenous to Australia, and has been revered by many cultures for its mitigating effects for a number of skin conditions, such as acne, eczema, athlete's foot, and the allergic reactions caused by insect bites. Tea tree has been naturalised just like all other plants, and grows all across the globe. The Body Shop manufactures tea tree products, such as face washes and creams, and sources them from the tea tree that grows on the foothills of Mount Kenya.

The reason tea tree oil is so effective against the development of acne is that it has antimicrobial properties as well. It thwarts the bacteria in their pursuit of sprouting new acne on the skin. However, tea tree oil is never used in its actual form, i.e., it is always diluted with a carrier oil, such as almond oil, before being applied topically on the skin. Despite the laundry list of benefits of tea tree oil, it is not recommended for prolonged use. It really depends on the genetics of the individual, as some people can tolerate the prolonged use of this oil, while others might start to show the emergence of allergic reactions. Tea tree oil is also used in creams that are specifically used for abatement of the sprouting of acne, and to pare down the prominence of blemishes left behind by acne.

Chapter 3
The Science of Plant Medicine

Phytochemistry and pharmacognosy are two key disciplines required for you to understand the science behind the working of the compounds present in the herbs. Phytochemistry is a subsidiary of botany that focuses on the study of phytochemicals, how they are produced in the plants, and how seasonal variations affect their concentrations. Pharmacognosy is an interdisciplinary field that has its epicentre in the medicinally important herbs, and discusses their extraction, and effects on human physiology. This chapter splays out the basics of these fields that form the bedrock for you to build your understanding of plant medicine.

Unveiling Phytochemistry: The Compounds Behind the Cure

Phytochemistry focuses on the biomolecules found in the plants. Before the 17th century, scientists focused on burning plants and examining the ash content, but found no results, as the ash content of poisonous and non-poisonous plants was found to be the same. Nicholas Leméry was the first prominent scientist who worked on extracting and determination of the phytochemicals present in plants, and made use of alcohol as a solvent for the extraction process. Robert Boyle lived in the same era, i.e., the 1600s, and was able to disprove Aristotle's theory that matter was composed of four elements. Boyle did not exactly know that alkaloids are the principal pharmacologically active compounds found in many plants, but he was moving in the right direction, as he treated opium with potassium carbonate and alcohol for the extraction process.

Until the early 1800s, nicotine became the first alkaloid to be isolated. The poisonous alkaloid found in *Strychnos toxifera*, strychnine, was also isolated. Strychnine has been used as arrow poison since ancient times. Morphine was also successfully isolated from opium. Nevertheless, it took another hundred years for scientists to put their focus on the actual biosynthetic pathways that take place in the plans. Structural elucidation of the phytochemicals and their stereochemical aspects that allow different isomers and polymorphs of the same molecule to have pronounced and different effects on the human body became the epicentre of all scientific research by the twentieth century. The enzymatic reactions of the biosynthetic pathways became a subject of interest among scientists, and plant biochemistry burgeoned into the expansive field that we see today.

The pharmacognosist focuses on only the pharmacologically active phytochemicals. To be pharmacologically active means to have pronounced effect on the physiologic processes and biochemical pathways. Alkaloids, glycosides, saponins, and tannins are all pharmacologically active compounds. Flavonoids straddle the midriff, and carbohydrates, fats, and proteins are of only dietetic importance.

Herbal Synergy: The Entourage Effect in Plant Medicine

According to research that has been conducted in the field of medicine, the biochemicals inside of the body work together to produce a remarkably pronounced effect that is greater than the additive effect of the individual biomolecules. This is not just true for the phytochemicals that are ingested into the body, but also the biosynthetic molecules that are produced endogenously within the body. The entourage effect makes it possible to accelerate the healing process of any disease. This is why most medications, even those that are not of plant origin, are taken together with other medications, as they potentiate the cell-signalling or physiologic mechanisms within the body.

However, this is not applicable to all the drugs, as some drugs inhibit the action of other drugs. For instance, captopril and ibuprofen have serious interaction, and therefore, you cannot take the two medications together. This is because NSAIDS (non-steroidal anti-inflammatory drugs), inclusive of ibuprofen, generally cause a decrease in renal function. This also decreases the secretion of vasodilating renal prostaglandins that are released into the bloodstream from the kidneys. Prostaglandins have a role to play in the antihypertensive effect that is triggered by the ACE (angiotensin-converting enzyme) inhibitors. ACE inhibitors include captopril among other drugs. Therefore, the net antihypertensive effect of ACE inhibitors is decreased if you take NSAIDs, like ibuprofen, with them. Herbal remedies need to follow the same caution. Therefore, always keep your doctor in the loop if you plan to take herbal remedies and have been on a drug regimen prescribed by your doctor.

Furanocoumarins found in grapefruit juice can alter the bioavailability of certain drugs. These coumarins have the ability to inactivate certain cytochrome P550 enzymes of the liver, particularly, CYP3A4 and CYP3A5. As a result, the drugs that are metabolised by these isozymes show a marked increase in concentration in the plasma, and their bioavailability is increased. Bergapten is another coumarin found in bergamot oil that has the same effect. However, there are other compounds in grapefruit juice that rather decrease the absorption of drugs from the gut, and therefore, this juice has unpredictable effects on the bioavailability of drugs. Certain unnamed compounds activate the efflux pump controlling p-glycoprotein-mediated transport across the microvilli of the small intestine. The efflux pump takes certain absorbed drugs back into the gut, thereby decreasing their absorption and bioavailability. Fexofenadine (Telfast®), Losartan (Cozaar®), and vinblastine (Velban®) are absorbed in lesser amounts if taken with grapefruit juice.

From Plant to Prescription: The Journey of Herbal Compounds

Drug discovery studies are conducted to look for new compounds that can be potential curative treatments for diseases that do not have a cure yet. Numerous techniques of analytical chemistry are used to characterise the medicinally useful phytochemicals and extract them. Characterisation of the formulation to be used as medication is done by microscopy techniques, as well and x-ray crystallography, nuclear magnetic resonance (NMR), and Fourier transform infrared spectroscopy (FTIR). Raman spectroscopy and Karl Fischer titration are newly developed techniques currently under the spotlight. Once the formulation is characterised, the polymorph or isomer of a molecule with the greatest therapeutic efficacy is tested in animal models, and then in human volunteers in clinical trials. Successful drug candidates enter the market to be prescribed by doctors.

Clinical Trials and Herbal Efficacy

Clinical trials are conducted on human subjects and classified into four distinct phases. the first three phases are done in volunteers. Phase one clinical trials clarify bring the toxicology profile of the drug to prominence. If the drug produces any potential toxic effects, the trial culminates at this point and the drug fails to receive FDA (Food and Drug Administration) approval. If the drug shows no toxic effects, the drug candidate is plunged into phase two, wherein the pharmacokinetic and pharmacodynamic effects of the drug are delineated. The pharmacodynamics of a drug refer to its mechanism of action, i.e., the way it triggers its physiologic and biochemical response in the body. It also includes the organ system effects that the drug produces in the body. The pharmacokinetics refer to the ADME of the drug, which is an acronym for the absorption, distribution, metabolism, and elimination of the drug.

Phase three of the clinical trial delves deeper into the metabolism and biotransformation of the drug that happens in the liver. The bioavailability of different dosage forms (tablets, capsules, injections) and the routes of administration (oral, parenteral, subcutaneous, etc.) are also studied in an intensive manner. The drug is then marketed and the healthcare practitioners are directed to give feedback about the drug response that they see i patients, This phase is called the post-marketing surveillance phase, or phase four, of clinical trials. Some adverse and side effects of the drugs come to surface that were not determined during the first three phases of the clinical trials.

Potential drug interactions are determined till phase three as well. Given the multitude of drugs and the wide variety of comorbidities found in patients, it is not possible to completely circumscribe the interactions between different drugs. Therefore, phase four focuses on massive cohorts of data that drive the complete detail of the functions of the drug to fruition. It takes years for the four phases of a clinical trial to reach successful point of completion. Too many data points are involved and statistical analysis of clinical trial data allows the full picture to be painted.

Chapter 4
Cultivating Your Herbal Garden

The process of dedicating yourself to herbal remedies starts with a complete revamp of your backyard. The soil needs to be the right pH that can sustain the growth of herbs, and the use of fertilisers is highly imperative to supply the right nutrition to your herbs. Fertilising is just as important as irrigating the backyard and providing enough sunlight without scorching the plants. The trick is to nourish your herbs with the right amount of sunlight, water, and minerals, so that they can grow in an unimpeded fashion and produce the herbs that are suitable for your consumption. Remember, as discussed before, seasonal variation can severely impact the concentration of the phytochemicals in the plants, so you need to keep this factor in mind when you think to plant a certain plant.

Getting Started: Planning Your Herbal Garden

Generally, the soil of your garden is primed for the growth of plants in early spring, as the soil gets free form the shackles of the ice that melts after the winters. However, the sowing season for plants depends on the species of the plants. Some plant species are to be sowed in early spring, and some have to be sowed later in the year. For instance, some plant seeds are sowed in summer, and even in late summer. So, you need to check the botanical detail of the plant that you want to grow in your garden. It is advisable to have raised beds for different species of the plants, as these beds are enclosed with concrete or brick walls that enable the soil to be treated differently for dissimilar species of plants. Irrigating the soil might be done in a general manner through sprinklers that you might have installed in your garden, or with the help of a hose. However, plants that require a little more water than the others can have adverse effects, as the water can leach and percolate through the soil. Fertilisers can also be used with relative tension-free mind, as you would know that the soil requirements of a particular plant are being met in a particular bed.

The United States is divided into hardiness zones depending on the climatic conditions of a region. If a particular plant is rated cold-hardy for zones four through nine, it would not survive in a colder zone. Therefore, you might want to keep some specific desirable plants off your list because they might not be able to survive in your zone. This is something that is beyond your control, so you can think about growing other useful herbs.

If two different species of plants have similar watering and sunlight exposure requirements, you can sow the seeds together in a single enclosure or bed. This is a preferable; strategy, as companion plants that grow in a single enclosure tend to pull more nitrogen from the air and into their stomatal pores. This optimises the process of photosynthesis. Also, more nitrogen around the soil helps with nitrogen fixation and more nitrates become available for absorption up the roots of the plants.

Making raised beds for your garden and enclosing the plants keep the soil healthy and the growth of weeds to a minimum. Raised beds would require some investment from your end, as you would need bricks and cement to make these durable enclosures. Alternatively, corrugated metal sheets can also be used if you are looking for a cost-effective approach to make your garden.

On the other hand, in-ground gardening technique can be utilised instead of raised beds. This technique creates a depression or a crater-like space that is below the level of your garden. You would need to supply less water to plants grown in these spaces, but the soil could become waterlogged due to the lack of open spaces. Also, the risk of contamination is higher, as soil aeration is also reduced. Weeds are also more likely to grow.

Vertical gardening is also a trend among gardening enthusiasts. It makes use of repurposed bottles and cans to be placed on the walls. Vines can also be used to embellish your garden, as they add to the aesthetic attribute of your space. Also, removing grass can make it easier for the plants to be grown. Grass can hinder the growth of the root system of certain plants, especially the plants that have very extensive root systems. Make sure that your soil does not have too much clay, as it con pose drainage problems. Waterlogged soil can easily allow unhindered growth of bacteria.

Choosing Herbs Based on Therapeutic Needs and Organic Gardening Practices

The climatic conditions of your region can prove to be a major limiting factor that can preclude the planting of potential herbs of your choice. Also, you need to consider growing only those herbs that you really need to grow in your garden, based on your necessities.

Organic gardening practices have become trendsetters in the realm of backyard gardening. People are no longer divorced from the harmful effects of chemical fertilisers and pesticides. The fact that all synthetic chemical fertilisers and pesticides are sourced from naturally-occurring materials means that you can make use of these materials to grow your plants. The pesticide cycloprothrin used for rice paddies, for instance, is a derivative of the naturally-occurring compound, called pyrethrin, found in chrysanthemum flowers. In fact, before the advent of chemical pesticides, crushed petals of the chrysanthemum flower used to be sprinkled on the soil, as this is an effective pesticide. The crushed petals ward-off many insects that would otherwise feed on your plants.

Organic pesticides also rule out the threat of chemical pesticides leaching into the soil and being absorbed up the roots of the plants. These pesticides get into the phloem sap of the plants through the xylem vessels. When consumed by humans, the harmful chemicals of the pesticide get into our bodies and accumulate in our organs. Some pesticides might also contain traces of heavy metals, namely, lead, cadmium, and mercury. These metals undergo a process of bioaccumulation that makes them nearly impossible to be removed from the human body. This poses a threat to neurological function, especially in growing children.

Pest Control: Natural Solutions for a Healthy Garden

There is a range of natural pesticides that you can use instead of chemical pesticides. The controversy surrounding the use of chemical pesticides has gravitated people toward the use of naturally sourced pest control methods that have zero impact on the environment and human health. Also, these natural pest control methods have been tried and tested to be effective against a range of pests, inclusive of aphids. You do not eve have to go for complex and intricate methods of planting chrysanthemum flowers or something else that evokes labor form your end. You can make use of the things that you already have in your house. For instance, making a spray from dish-washing soap has been proven to be a very effective strategy to drive away pests. Adding vinegar to this concoction potentiates its pesticide property, which can be even further augmented by adding pepper oil.

The Timing of Harvesting Your Herbs and Methods of Preservation

As discussed in the previous chapters, seasonal variations have a pronounced effect on the phytochemical concentration found in your plants. You have to plan in advance about the sowing of seeds of each herb, so that you take into account the right sowing season and the season that can have the maximum concentration of the phytochemical in the herb. This strategy can help you attain cognisance of the seasonal time that can make the herb bear its maximum concentration of the phytochemicals.

Furthermore, you need to harvest the herb starting from the leaves, and pluck the lower leaves first, because they brown out as their age progresses. Place the herbs in sealed mason jars in the refrigerator, so that the smell of the other items in the fridge does not get absorbed into the herbs. Afterwards, air-dry the herbs by hanging them. The other way to preserve herbs is to freeze them. You can use these herbs by adding them to butter, and you can also make herb-infused vinegar. For extraction, place the herbs in a jar and pour any kind of alcohol into it, and let the jar stand for five to six weeks. You will get a concentrated extract. For instance, you can add vodka to a jar of vanilla beans in this way.

Chapter 5

Harvesting and Storing Your Bounty

Herbs are subject to a change in the phytochemical concentration that are presided over by seasonal variations. You might find a high concentration of the preferred phytochemical in a particular season that gradually decreases to a lower value after a few weeks. This might prove to be a slight inconvenience for you, especially of you wanted to have a more potent harvest. The timing of your harvest plays a very important role owing to this reason. Handling the herbs is the next important step that must be done right in order for you to be able to keep the herb intact. Preserving the herbs for later use, or making an extract right away depends entirely on your own volition. There are some common mistakes and pitfalls that must be avoided when you dedicate yourself to this process.

The Art of Timing: When to Harvest Your Herbs

The timing must be considered when you decide to grow your herbal garden. The sowing of seeds is a process that can allow a bit of flexibility, so that you can have a few days of harvesting well into the period when the phytochemicals can reach a bit higher concentration. Each herb has its own unique sowing period and harvesting period, and these must be taken into account when you commit yourself to this process. The plant might not stay firm if you wait to long for harvest, so you need to harvest the herb at its allocated time with a little flexibility, as you cannot prolong its life span.

Harvesting Techniques: Doing It Right

There are certain rules for annual and perennial plants, nut there are certain plants that do not fit in these categories. The advantage with growing herbs is that they mature quickly as compared to most other edible plants. Most other plants have to mature and bolt to produce flowers that then turn into fruits. With herbs, you need to flowers, and even if the plant produces flowers on the stems, they can be pruned carefully without damaging the stem.

Pruning and harvesting are synonymous for herbs, as opposed to most other plants. Pruning must be done, but it must be done in a careful manner not to cut too much foliage. Cutting excessive foliage actually encourages healthy overall growth of the plant. Also, it helps the plant to maintain good shape. Fast-growing herbs, like basil, the Indian dill, and cilantro, require regular pruning to maintain optimum growth. The same is also done for slow-growing perennial plants. Perennial plants are those that have a life-span of more than two years, while annual plants last for only one season.

Even if the annual plants have a life span of only one season, never deracinate the entire plant when you have to harvest the leaves of the herbs. You must wait for the killing frost to arrive and for the plant to die out naturally. Perennials tend to form woody stems, and you must be careful when you prune these herbs. The wooden stem is from where the shoots grow out, and is rich in phloem and xylem vessels that supply nutrition to the entire plant. Cutting into the woody stems can damage the plant and retard the growth of new shoots.

The first harvest is always meager in amount, but consistent harvesting and pruning of limited foliage can help you attain bigger harvests as time progresses. Harvesting the plant must be done when it is dry. Snipping wet foliage results in bacterial contamination of the plant. Also, for your final harvest, if you are cutting the entire stem, try making a slanted cut, as this helps the stem to grow into new shoots quickly. As far as the timing of the day is concerned, harvest your plant between mid-morning and early afternoon, as this time of that day allows most herbs to be packed with the highest concentration of essential oils. Also, the most fragrant phytochemicals are rich in the herbs in the time-frame, giving your harvest a very potent scent.

Generally, the appearance of the herbs gives you a good indication about the timing of the harvest. If any of the annual herbs are drooping and appearing limp, it is time to harvest. For the perennials, if you notice flowers growing out of the stems, it is time for the harvest. The pruning or harvesting or process is done in a proper fashion to allow quick growing of the stem and the leaves.

For snipping the stem, do not cut more than one-third of the entire stem. Also, allow adequate pruning after snipping the stem, as this helps the plant to grow quickly. When pruning a small part of the stem, do it about one-fourth of an inch above the leaf node. The cut is made at an angle to the transverse plane, i.e., also called a slanted cut or an angled cut.

Post-Harvest Handling, Drying, and Storage

Post-harvest handling is done the right way to prolong the storage time of your herbs. You can put the herbs in sealed mason jars and place them in the refrigerator. There are two main methods of handling the herbs. They are either air-dried or frozen to maintain prolonged longevity of the herbs. Air-drying can be done by hanging them from a spot on the beams of your house, or any other place from where they can be hung vertically. This manner of air-drying gives your house a good rustic look, and since air flows freely through the foliage, it spreads the scent of the herbs throughout the house.

The other way is to freeze the herbs. Freezing allows quick drying of the herbs and prolong the life span of the herbs. Also, they can be stored for even longer periods of time if they are frozen, as freezing slows down the speed of chemical reactions. Decomposition is a chemical reaction that slows as well, hence prolonging the life of your herbs.

Organising Your Home Apothecary Stock

The organisation of your herbal stock is a process that makes it easier for you to choose the right herbs in times of need. You can place the herbs in beautiful glass bottles or mason jars. Labelling the jars is important, as everyone in your house may not be familiar with the appearance of the herbs. You need to label the jars with paper that can be pasted on the glass. Also, you can write the date of harvest, so that you would know when a particular stock of herbs would start to go off.

Overcrowding is a common mistake that must be avoided when growing herbs, as it does not allow the herbs to grow a healthy root system. Roots need much pace beneath the soil, and if you are growing too many herbs in a small area, their root systems would compete for nutrients and space.

Allowing the herb to blossom is another common mistake, as many people like to see the flowers embellish the garden. However, the fact that flowers start to bloom is an indication that the plant is about to complete its life cycle. Luckily, this is an avoidable death, and you only need to pinch the flower off the plant. This way, your plant will thrive incessantly. Thus, never allow the flower to turn into seed.

Pruning must be done on a regular basis, and always look for necrotised and brown foliage on the plant. If you do, snip it off, as this will prevent the spread of the dead tissue.

Chapter 6

Herbal Remedies for Everyday Ailments

There are many products on the shelves of the pharmacy that are herbal remedies. The chief phytochemicals of medicinal importance have been listed in all major pharmacopeia since centuries, and now we have advanced chemistry techniques to synthesise the compounds of pharmacological importance. Pharmaceutical sciences have undergone substantial growth that allow the relevant polymorph and of the molecule to be studied extensively. The breakthroughs in pharmaceutical technology allows the most efficient drug delivery systems to be used for the delivery of these synthetic compounds into the body. These formulations manufactured by pharmaceutical companies have excipients that maximise the bioavailability of the drug. Although the herbs that you would use would not allow a quick recovery from an ailment, they can be used occasionally to help the body augment its physiologic functioning. Still, you can use these herbs as an alternative to the over-the-counter drugs that are available without a prescription at the pharmacy.

Nature's Medicine Cabinet: An Overview

The herbs that you grow in your garden can be used to slow down the progression of the disease that you are suffering from. Common respiratory and gastric illnesses can be alleviated using these herbs that have the relevant phytochemicals packed in raw form. Although these herbs, by no means, serve as a substitute to the over-the-counter medication that you must use to recuperate completely from your illness, they can be used to provide a synergistic effect. The collective healing effect of the medicines and the herbs can help you recover from the disease. Also, using herbs can help you feel better as well, as the aroma of the herbs has a natural uplifting characteristic.

Natural Solutions for Stress and Anxiety

It is not only the ailments that warrant the use of the herbs that you have grown in your garden. Essential oils that you get from these herbs can be used for many purposes that are not related to recovering from a disease. For instance, eucalyptus oil can be used by those who suffer from insomnia, as the essential oil helps to mellow the senses and helps slide the user into a state of deep sleep. Eucalyptus oil is a natural anxiolytic and sedative that relieves the nerves and induces a state of sleep. Calming the nerves is a indispensable property of eucalyptus oil.

Preparing eucalyptus oil from eucalyptus oil is a very easy process that can be followed quickly.

Preparation of Eucalyptus Oil

You would need a carrier oil that has the purpose of a vehicle, i.e., it serves a medium in which the eucalyptus oil can be absorbed and carried into the body. Almond oil is a good carrier oil that can be used for this purpose. You can buy almond oil form a good pharmacy and there are many good brands. First off, you need to wash the eucalyptus herbs in water in a dish. Let them dry in open air, so that the water does not mix with the oil and hinder the process.

Industrial and laboratory processes of extraction of volatile oils are highly intricate and cannot be done at home. They require the use of advanced techniques, instruments, and reagents. Supercritical fluid extraction and solid phase micro-extraction are two processes that have gained monumental traction over the years and are under intensive research. Methyl polysiloxane solid phase micro-extraction is done for eucalyptus leaves that gathers the volatile oils in the headspace above the leaves when the process is done at 37 degree Celsius for 10 minutes. The fibers of methyl polysiloxane absorb the oils, which are then desorbed at 200 degree Celsius before analysis through capillary gas chromatography. The method of extraction of the volatile oil presides over the composition of the volatile oil. The eucalyptus oil that is extracted in this manner has a composition that is different from that of steam-distilled eucalyptus oil. Nevertheless, you can get a somewhat suitable collection of the oil if you do it using carrier oils.

The process of letting the oil and other constituents leach into the carrier oil is called maceration. You need to pulverise the eucalyptus herbs using a pestle and mortar that can be bought from the nearest pharmacy. Alternatively, you can simply crush the herbs using your hands. Next, steep the herbs into a bowl containing the carrier oil. The process of pulverisation allows the plant cells to break and release their constituents. Maceration and steeping the crushed herbs into a carrier oil allows the constituents to absorb into the oil. Macerating the herbs for up to six weeks allows the constituents to be maximally absorbed into the oil.

This eucalyptus oil can then be used for a range of applications. This includes using it on your pillows when you go to bed. The oil releases a powerful and fragrant odor that helps insomniacs fall asleep quickly. The calming effect on the nerves slides you into a stress-free state of mind.

Natural Solutions for Digestive Health

Your garden can be a source of producing castor oil that has been used for digestive health for centuries. Its main purpose is to be used as a laxative for patients who have constipation. Additionally, it is also used for patients who need to undergo a surgery for which the bowels must be empty, so the castor oil is given to such patients that helps them to clear their bowels.

Castor oil is given to patients of constipation by mouth. It is only given in very small doses, as a small dose of the oil is enough to produce very strong peristaltic movements. Also, castor oil is an emetic, and causes retching and vomiting if given in large amounts, so consideration must be given to this attribute of castor oil. large doses can also cause diarrhoea. Castor oil is broken down in the intestines to release ricinoleic acid, the principal component driving the laxative effect. This fatty acid gets absorbed into the intestines and evokes strong smooth muscle contractions of the small intestine.

Natural Solutions for Skincare

Tea tree oil has many antimicrobial properties that makes it ideal for the treatment of acne. The oil can be applied to the acne before diluting it with a carrier oil, such as almond oil. However, some people with nodular acne can also apply tea tree oil directly on the acne, thus mitigating the replication of the bacteria that drive the growth of acne.

Aloe vera has a laundry list of benefits of benefits for the skin. Aloe vera is mostly made up of water, and the gel can be easily collected by breaking the plant. If you happen to develop a rash on your skin, the gel can be applied directly on the skin to mollify the affected area. The application of aloe vera gel makes the skin supple and prevents the bacteria from multiplying on the skin. people prone to acne can find aloe vera gel very useful.

Neem oil can be extracted in the same way that has been described for eucalyptus oil. Neem is a herb that is indigenous to the Indian subcontinent. The herb has very powerful; cleansing effect on the skin, and people with nodular acne find it extremely useful as a successful remedy to completely eradicate the acne form their skin. The oil can clarify skin tone as well.

Natural Solution for Boosting Immune Health

Astragalus is a well-known herb that is used in Chinese medicine to boost immune health. Apart from this, guduchi is another herb that has undergone extensive research. Guduchi is also known as giloy, and has the binomial name, *Tinospora cordifolia*. Guduchi has a potent immunomodulating effect that boosts the immune system and helps the white blood cells fight an infection. The herb underwent clinical research trials during COVID-19 pandemic, and showed promise in bolstering the immune system of the patients afflicted by coronavirus.

Echinacea and oregano have immunomodulating activity as well. Though not so potent immunomodulators as the aforementioned herbs, these can be consumed on a daily basis to help augment the capability of your immune system. Oregano is added as a condiment and flavouring to many foods, and has a flagrant aroma that makes the dish taste even better. Turmeric has immune boosting properties as well, and is a very popular condiment that is added to a range of dishes to make the final product taste and smell great. Turmeric powder can be added to a variety of foods and in marinades. The marinating property of turmeric makes delicious foods. Turmeric is also an essential herb used in Chinese medicine.

Ginseng has been used in many energy drinks, but it also has the ability to boost the immune system. The active compounds that contribute to this effect are called ginsenosides, and these compounds can make the immune system work more efficiently. It is also used to heighten energy levels and decrease fatigue. Also, it can elevate the mood.

Chapter 7
The Art of Herbal Preparation

Taking your herbs and subjecting them to treatment procedures that turn them into useful remedies is something that you must be accustomed to in order to effectively make use of your herb garden. This chapter helps you find ways to effectively transform your raw herbal stock into extracts that can be used to make tinctures, salves, potions, and poultices. The art of the apothecary is something that used to be a skill worth acquiring in the olden times. Every household had a member that was adept at using herbs and making extracts out of them. Salves and poultices were the only way to alleviate pain and treat wounds and infections, so it was a skill that was highly revered. Every town or village had an apothecary who had the expertise to treat patients, but it was encouraged to have someone in every household who can make poultices and potions without the help of an expert apothecary.

Mastering Herbal Concoctions and Infusions

Making herbal infusions is the most common way of consuming the herbs that you grow in your garden. Teas are the most famous form of infusions that are fairly dominant across the globe. Infusions are made by a process of maceration, i.e., by steeping the herbs into a utensil containing hot water. The period for which the herbs are allowed to infuse into the water varies for different kinds of infusions. The strength of the infusion is determined by the period of time that the herbs stays in the medium that soaks its oils and constituents. Any medium other than water can be used, and this medium is called the menstruum. The greater the time the herbs are soaked in the menstruum, the greater the amount of the plant constituents that get soaked into the menstruum, resulting in a stronger infusion. Tea is a rather weak infusion because the herbal content is soaked for a limited amount of time in the water.

Generally, leaves are infused for four hours. The flowers require half as much time, i.e., two hours. Seeds are infused for 30 minutes, and the same time is utilised for berries.

You can determine the strength of the infusion by taking a look at its color. Stronger infusions have darker color, because the anthocyanins present in the herbs that give them their characteristic colours get absorbed in greater amounts if you let the herbs get soaked in the menstruum for longer periods of time. This makes infusions more enjoyable among herb enthusiasts as compared to pills and tablets.

The infusions have uses that go beyond your own personal use. For instance, an infusion of garlic and cayenne can ward off rodents, such as rabbits. This infusion can be sprayed onto your plants to keep rabbits away, which normally find every opportunity to gnaw at your precious herbal plants. The infusions can also be used in the salves that you keep for personal use. Infusions can be stored for up to two weeks in the refrigerator.

Making Aloe Vera Infusion

Aloe vera has the ability to reduce rashes that appear on your skin. The redness and swelling subsides after the application of aloe vera gel that can be squeezed out of the pulp that you find in aloe vera gel. However, the pulp can also be used to make infusions of aloe vera. The infusions can be consumed to improve gastric health, especially in patients of constipation. The infusion is also given to patients of irritable bowel syndrome (IBS) and ulcerative colitis. The process of making the infusion is simple. Dried aloe vera is placed in a jar that contains alcohol, and macerated for six weeks. You can add crushed calendula flower to the infusion as well.

The Difference Between Extracts and Tinctures

Tinctures are made using the same methods as used for extracts. However, tinctures are made by using a bigger stock of the herbs that is placed in the same amount of alcohol. This gives a very concentrated extract of the herb, which is called a tincture.

Making a Decoction

Decoction are simply potent infusions that are made by heating. The herb and the water are placed in a saucepan and brought to a simmer. The resulting mixture is strained, and poured into a jar.

Medicinal Uses of Herbal Extracts, Infusions, and Tinctures

Peppermint is used for making infusions that can be consumed to relieve an upset stomach. The constituents of peppermint get dissolved in the water and provide relief form abdominal pain and cramps. Flatulence also gets relieved to a particular extent. Peppermint is also added to yogurt and consumed with food that put a lot of workload on the stomach, such as cheesy meat steaks. This makes the meal easy to be digested by the stomach.

Thyme contains an oil called thymol, which makes thyme very useful as an antiseptic. The infusion made with thyme can be used to fight halitosis, i.e., bad breath. The antiseptic property of the infusion makes it useful for mouth sores as well. Laryngitis is an inflammation of the throat that also calls for the use of thyme infusion due to its antiseptic action.

Chamomile has the same uses as lavender, as it is a sedative and an anxiolytic. The infusion made with chamomile can be ingested to relieve the senses and imbue calm. The effects are not as potent as an infusion of lavender, but can be used as a substitute when you run out of lavender.

Sage is a herb that stands out in its family of herbs, as it not a good condiment. the infusion made from it is useful as a potent anti-inflammatory, and can be used to relieve sore throat. Sage also improves cognitive health and boosts memory. You might also try making a tincture from sage and use it for joint pain, as it might alleviate the pain to a certain degree.

Making Herbal Capsules and Powders

Making powders from herbs is an easy process. All you need is a pestle and a mortar to get started. Even if you do not have a pestle and a mortar, you can sue your coffee grinder to pulverise the herbs. It os best to buy a new coffee grinder for the purpose of pulverising the herbs and turning them into a powder. This is because the coffee would get mixed with the herbs and the fragrant smell of the herbs could get diminished to a significant degree.

For herbal capsules, all you need to do is buy empty gelatine capsules. These are the same capsules that are used to encapsulate pharmaceutical powders. Put the herbal powder that you have prepared in a bowl with a wide diameter, and slide the capsules through the powders to fill the capsules. This gives you filled capsules that can be used for the desired purpose.

Making Herbal Syrups and Elixirs

Herbal syrups are made from decoctions. Decoctions serve as the base of the syrup to which honey or sugar is added. the natural anti-bacterial property of honey helps to preserve the herbal syrup and prolong its shelf-life, since bacterial contamination and decomposition of the syrup is minimised. Adding honey or sugar also amplifies the palatability of the syrup, as sweet herbal syrups are gracefully accepted by children. Also, you can add carbonated water to the syrup to make herbal soda.

Herbal elixirs are made by a combination of herbs, honey, and alcohol. A stress relieving elixir can be made from astragalus, ashwagandha, and basil. The three herbs can be pulverised in a coffee grinder, and placed in a jar to which honey can be added. You can take half cup of each herb. Sugar is also taken in the same amount, i.e., half cup. Two and a half cups of alcohol are then added to this mixture. The herbs are allowed to be infused for almost two weeks. The elixir can be stored in a cool and dark place where the elixir can stay active for several years.

Chapter 8

Herbal Recipes and Formulations

The primary benefit of growing your own herbal garden is to be able to have access to a wide variety of herbal concoctions that have been tailor-made for each kind of ailment. You can reduce your reliance on the pharmaceuticals that are typically available in the market. It has been a growing and popular trend to shift away from the undeniable reliance on pharmaceuticals and to gravitate back toward nature. This is why herbal concoctions and remedies have resurfaced. Dependence on processed foods and ready-to-eat meals has also become the subject of stigma owing to the laundry list of harmful effects that these foods can have on your health. Herbal remedies are just a part of the equation that helps to redeem yourself and break free of the shackles of the scourge of processed food.

The rise in autism spectrum disorders and autoimmune disorder has become the subject of recent speculation and all fingers point toward the overuse of processed food and ready-to-eat meals. The advances of the twentieth century have made life considerable easier for us, but also made us susceptible to a range of diseases that have had a very low incidence in the past century. Celiac disease, which arises due to allergy to gluten, has also seen a spike in cases. All in all, it has become a necessary trend to shift toward healthy living practices to lower the occurrence of these diseases in the human population.

Specialized Formulations for Immune Support

Turmeric

You can grow your own turmeric in your garden to help create formulations that can boost immune health. Turmeric powder can be produced in the same manner that has been discussed in the preceding chapter. Capsules can be created from the powder, and these capsules can be taken whenever someone in the house contracts an infectious respiratory disease. Turmeric has immunomodulating and anti-inflammatory phytochemicals that can alleviate sore throat to a certain degree.

Turmeric is also undergoing substantial research on its impact on autoimmune disorders. The powder might produce symptomatic relief in the volunteers who have been recruited for the clinical trials, but it is too early to have a say about this. However, the fact that turmeric has a powerful impact on the immune system cannot be overlooked.

Echinacea

Echinacea has been a subject of numerous studies conducted by the National Center for Complementary and Integrative Health (NCCIH). This auxiliary of the National Institutes of Health (NIH) has found that echinacea has a profound impact on the duration of the cold and flu that afflicts the patients. The herb can provide symptomatic relief for sore throat and cough, and reduce the number of days for which the patient remains incapacitated by the illness. If you have contracted cold or the flu, the best way to take this herb is in the form of infusions that can either be gargled or consumed. The remedy is to be taken at least three times a day. However, always consult your doctor before taking any herbal treatment along with the medication that has been prescribed to you for a swift recovery.

Ginger

Ginger has its own advantages when used as a remedy for infectious diseases. The compounds that drive its anti-inflammatory, and anti-oxidant effect are gingerol and shogaol. These compounds have been shown to prevent the progression of respiratory syncytial virus (RSV) to a substantial degree. Regular consumption of ginger can protect against a number of diseases. The phytochemicals present in ginger help to protect against a number of diseases.

Cinnamon

Cinnamon is well-known among the masses for a number of benefits that it imparts to its user. It is an anti-oxidant, and retards the rates of aging process of the body by combating the action of free radicals that are produced as reactive oxygen species. By inhibiting the action of reactive oxygen species, the compounds present in cinnamon protect against a number of diseases that result from inflammation. Cinnamaldehyde is the principal component of cinnamon that drives its anti-inflammatory action.

Peppermint

This herb is a cross between water mint and spearmint, and boasts the properties of both of these herbs. it has a potent anti-oxidant effect that helps to mop up the free radicals inside of your body. People even feel refreshed and rejuvenated after consuming peppermint or peppermint derived foods. Menthol is a phytochemical found in it that gives it the cooling effect that you get after consuming it. Menthol is also added to other products, such as shampoos, which gives a cooling effect on your scalp. Head & Shoulders has a shampoo in its product line that has menthol added to it.

Peppermint can also be inhaled into the body through the nostrils, and it has a soothing effect on the nasal passages. The bronchodilating effect of menthol makes peppermint a useful herb that can be inhaled by patients of cold and the flue. It helps to dilate the bronchi and allows greater passage of air into the lungs.

Formulations for Anxiety Relief That Induce Sleep

Lemon Balm

This is a herb that is well-known among those who find it difficult to fall asleep. Lemon balm has been the key ingredient in herbal tea blends that allow the user to fall asleep quickly. Growing this herb should be done with extreme prudence, especially if you reside in a mild climate in the United States. This is because the herb tends to undergo aggressive growth and spread that can be hard to control. Lemon balm helps to improve the mood as well, so you can drink it in small amounts throughout the day to feel lively and vibrant without the fear of feeling overly drowsy.

Catnip

This herb is renowned for being used by cats, as it gives them a feeling of intoxication similar to what humans get after a dose of psychedelic drugs. Without causing any intoxicating effect, catnip can be added to concoctions containing lemon balm to produce a sedating effect for the user. It is only used in this way, i.e., to potentiate the anxiolytic and sedative effect of other herbs.

Making a Poultice

The herbs that are renowned for their anti-inflammatory and healing effects have been used for making poultices for centuries. Turmeric and ginger are the prime ingredients for making a poultice. Since a poultice is especially used for healing wounds, the ingredients are specifically chosen on the basis of helping the wound to seal. The following ingredients are used:

- Almost one teaspoon of turmeric
- Finely chopped ginger
- One garlic clove that has been freshly chopped
- One quarter of chopped onion
- Two teaspoons of coconut oil
- Cotton bandage

The coconut oil is to be added to a saucepan and the rest of the ingredients are also added in tandem. The whole thing is heated until it is dry. The dried poultice is added to a bowl and allowed to cool off until it does not scald your skin. A cloth or large bandage is placed flat and the poultice is placed at the center. The cloth is then folded and the poultice applied to the affected area.

Chapter 9
Herbalism in Daily Life

The art of making and using herbs helps to develop a lifestyle that drifts you away from the unrelenting reliance on allopathic medications. Humans have succumbed to the breakthroughs of the modern world, so much so that we do not even realise that there are certain attributes of the modern technology that can make us sick. Integrating herbalism and reliance on nature actually creates a wholesome opportunity for us to bring back the ways of our ancestors and resurrect the ancient practices that are starting to fade into oblivion. The advantages that herbalism offers are innumerable, and brings you closer to a holistic wellness strategy that supports your overall physical, mental, and spiritual health.

Everyday Herbalism: Making It a Lifestyle

Indubitably, the advances of modern medicine have an indefatigable influence on the healthcare system. Yes, there are many diseases that call for intricate attention of doctors, but certain common illnesses of the gastrointestinal tract and respiratory system can be treated with herbs that have proven effects that mitigate the spread of disease and provide symptomatic relief.

You can start your day with herbal teas that can help you feel more energetic and free of toxins that build up in side of the human body over the course of the day. There are many teas that can be consumed to help you cleanse your blood. The anthocyanins and flavonoids make you feel more energetic and free of toxins. Hibiscus tea and other popular teas can help start your day with a clean blood circulatory system.

Of course, the only way you can utilise the maximum effects of these herbal teas and tonic is to have a correct sleep pattern. Going to bed early and getting up early in the morning helps regulates the endocrine system that controls the secretion of hormones. A bad sleep pattern can minimize your chances of reaching your maximum potential, as you are not exposed to sunlight that lights up the horizon at daybreak. All living things perform better if they get exposed to sunlight on a daily basis through a correct sleep pattern.

Herbs in Nutrition and Cooking

Herb-infused oils can be used for cooking. They lend a great taste to the meal that you cook and the taste of the meal can be augmented even further by garnishing the dish with herbs. You do not even have to limit yourself when you use the culinary oil that has been infused with the herb. Such culinary oils can be used for all types of cooking, from baking pizzas to sautéing bread. One such example is rosemary oil, *Rasmarinus officinalis.* rosemary oil gives a great fragrant smell to the meals that you cook, and it can also be added to your shampoo to make it even better smelling than before. Rosemary has the benefit of reducing the dandruff on the scalps of those who are susceptible to it, and also diminishes the problem of itching to a substantial degree.

Dried herbs are used to make herb-infused oils. This reduces the risk of bacterial contamination and the emergence of the bacterium that cause botulism, *Clostridium botulinum.* This bacterium is the driving factor of botulism. Herbs that are commonly added to culinary oils include oregano (*Origanum vulgare*), ginger (*Zingiber officinale*), garlic (*Allium sativum*), and a wide variety of cayenne (*Capsicum* spp.). You would need a Crockpot and sterilise the container into which you need to pour the oil. If there is no sterilisation method available, wash the container or bottle thoroughly and dry it in the sun. There should be no moisture left in this container or bottle. Waxed paper would also be needed for this crockpot method. Carrier oils of choice are also need to make the herb-infused cooking oil.

Making Herb-Infused Cooking Oil by the Stovetop Infusion Method

First off, a warm infusion is made using the ratio method that makes use of correct ratios of herbs and the oil. the following steps have to be followed:

Take a container that has been sterilised or thoroughly cleaned. Add one ounce of the herb and ten ounces of the oil at room temperature.

Use a clean spoon to mix and place a waxed paper on the top of the jar before sealing it with the lid. This keeps the oil safe from the chemicals that might be present on the lid's inner surface.

Roll the jar to let the contents be mixed in a thorough fashion. Place this jar in a dark and dry cabinet to let the herbs infuse into the oil for up to a period of six weeks.

Use a funnel that has been lined with cheesecloth on the inner side and another jar into which the infusion can be filtered. The herbs are to be squeezed as much as possible, so that the oil can be harvested to a maximum degree. Compost the herbs that remain behind. You can add vitamin E to slow down the oxidation of the oil.

Now the sealed jars are to be heated in a water bath in a saucepan for six to eight hours at 140 degree Fahrenheit that has been almost one quarter filled with water. Keep a watchful eye on the amount of water in the saucepan, and top it up as the water boils off.

Strain the oil and label it for use in cooking.

Nighttime Rituals With Herbs

The body's natural circadian rhythm presides over your timing of sleep. The circadian rhythm is naturally wired to make the body feel that it needs to rest and recover at night through a time-frame that is dedicated to sleep. Your body undergoes tissue repair when it is resting and when you go to sleep. Many people suffer from an inability to sleep at the right time at night, or to have the luxury to sleep at all. The circadian rhythm is also called the body clock, and makes you feel drowsy and imbues the tendency to fall asleep at night. People who have disturbed sleep patterns tend to go late to bed and wake up late in the morning. The circadian rhythm gets upset and the hormonal balance also goes off the even keel. A galore of pathological problems take birth if the circadian rhythm remains upset. Therefore, it is better to resolve the issue and nip the problem in its bud before it blooms into a full-blown predicament.

There are some prescription drugs, called hypnotics, that have become the most commonly prescribed drugs in the world. These include Ambien® (zolpidem) among other drugs to which people have become addicted to an extent that they cannot possibly imagine to go to sleep without taking these drugs. Though these drugs are safe, it is better to get yourself free from the clutches of these drugs and the pharmaceutical companies manufacturing and selling these drugs. A nighttime ritual can be designed in such a way that your body slides into a state of relaxation and tranquility.

When the time approaches for you to go to bed, take a bath. If you have winters in your region, take a warm bath, as it calms the senses and initiates a relaxed state of mind. Meditate and allow the mind to calm down. If you are married, your partner and yourself can massage each other. Drink warm milk, and use herbal essential oils to sleep. Lavender oil can be dropped directly on your pillow in two to three drops. The aroma that it gives off helps you to go to sleep quickly. Also, try to do all of this at the right time, i.e., early at night, so that your body's circadian rhythm kicks into action and helps you fall asleep quickly, thus maximising the effects of the essential oil and your nighttime routine.

Teaching Herbalism to Family and Friends

The best thing to do is to spread the awareness of herbal medicine to your family and friends, so that they follow suit and put on the same shoes. The way mankind has become hooked to drugs has set off an alarm that cannot be ignored, and nonchalance can only stand in the way of you realizing the full extent of your journey into the realm of herbal medicine. Bringing your loved ones and friends into the fold of herbalism can make herbal practices undergo aggressive expansion. This also helps people to return to the ways of their forefathers who used to be adept at farming and animal husbandry practices. Cultivating your own garden and using the produce to uplift your life can make you feel empowered.

Spreading herbal knowledge and the olden ways that have shaped mankind is a good way to feel better about yourself. Knowledge is power, and in the hands of the majority, it can drive change. Pharmaceutical companies tout their finished pharmaceutical products (FFPs) and boast about their advantages, but all these drugs have a downside that manifests in the form of side effects. With herbal remedies, there is no downside, and you can reap all the advantages without getting exposed to any side effects.

Chapter 10
Mind, Body, and Spirit

Herbal remedies have the advantage of not just uplifting your physical health, but also your mental and emotional well-being. Your mental and emotional well-being are targeted by allopathic medicine as well, but individual drugs do not have the capability to uplift your emotional state while ramping up a physiologic process at the same time. This is where herbal remedies overtake modern medicine, as herbal remedies might not be as potent, but they target your physical, emotional, and mental state simultaneously. This holistic approach has enabled herbal remedies to gain traction over the years and become a dominant force.

The Holistic Philosophy of Herbalism

The holistic philosophy of herbalism is grounded in the fact that the entire body is an interconnected system and that these systems cannot be treated separately. When you subjugate the body to the effects of a herb, the herb produces its effects on all of these systems. This is especially true if you try to think about how herbal remedies work and the feeling that you get from using them. You can feel the effects of the herbs o your emotional state and mood as well. The mood-enhancing effect cannot be overlooked, and your mental status also experiences an improvement.

Some patients need holistic therapeutic measures to address their concerns. For example, patients suffering form post-traumatic stress disorder (PTSD) experience multi-pronged pain that encompasses physical, mental, and emotional well-being. When they recall the traumatic experiences that they had to go through, the synapses make connection in their minds and their pain receptors get activated to send the same nerve impulses. Their mental status remains afflicted with the same events, as these events play again and again like a tape recorder on repeat. Their emotional status takes the toll form this experience, as they lose trust in people in general, and start to look at everything through the lens of skepticism. Such patients benefit greatly from herbal therapies. They can feel better if they inhale lavender oil or chamomile oil. The anxiolytic effect of these herbs calms their senses, and instills a sense of peace and tranquility.

The philosopher, Hippocrates, is considered the father of medicine, and laid down the foundation for holistic therapies. The oath that doctors take before graduating is also the one that Hippocrates crafted during his time, and all healers were supposed to take the oath prior to formally assuming the obligations of the healer. It is called the

Hippocratic oath. Chinese medicine and Ayurvedic medicine absorbed the teachings of Hippocrates as well, and considers the body an interconnected system that must be treated wholly in order to treat a person that is sick.

War heroes who have had their limbs or parts of limbs amputated undergo a kind of pain called the phantom pain. It makes the person feel that the amputated body part is still there. The pain is relieved with pain killers such as NSAIDs, but the emotional and mental toll that the person takes does not get treated with drugs like ibuprofen. Such patients need to be settled into the new norm, and they are given holistic health therapies, such as Tai Chi, yoga, and meditation. Herbal health is also a holistic therapy, and essential oil, like lavender, chamomile, and lemon balm can ease the hardship of such patients. Victims of sexual assault experience pelvic floor dysfunction, and tremors due to the horror that they went through. They are also encouraged to meditate and be subjected to holistic therapies to make them feel better and to get back to a normal life.

Spiritual and Meditative Uses of Herbs

The notion of embarking on a spiritual journey into the depths of the inner self is deeply ingrained in Ayurvedic medicine, which is the oldest of all health systems. When using some of the herbs to meditate, you need to be sure that these herbs do not provoke an allergic reaction in you. If they do, discontinue their use immediately. Below you can find some herbs that have been used to gain an insight into spirituality.

Kava

This plant's leaves are used as ritual tea in the Pacific islands. it has been a famous tea to relieve the symptoms of anxiety. it has its action on GABAergic neurotransmission in the neuraxis, which gives you a feeling of sedation and a relief from anxiety. This is the same mechanism of action that we see with drugs called benzodiazepines, which include alprazolam (Xanax®). GABA (gamma-aminobutyric acid) is an inhibitory neurotransmitter and benzodiazepines and kava potentiates its action, making the person who consumes this herb or the drugs to be subject to a state of somnolence. Anxiety is also relieved. The best way to take the herb is to use its leaves to make tea. Meditation that is done afterward becomes easier to perform, as the nerves become subjugated by a sense of tranquility.

Sage

Sage can also be used to calm the senses. The research that has been conducted on this herb has been shown to alleviate anxiety and induce sleep.

Chamomile

Chamomile has little scientific evidence to support the idea that it induces a sense of calm and relief from anxiety. That is why there has been limited focus on the extraction or synthesis of the essential oil. However, you can consume it by making tea. It is the best way to take the herb.

Hawthorn

This is a herb that has been used since olden times to lower blood pressure. Hawthorn has attributes that go beyond only physically healing the heart, as it is used for emotionally healing the heart as well. The herb has beautiful flowers that are used when someone has to mend the heart of the one that they have hurt. It has also been used to express the feelings of love for someone.

Rauwolfia

This plant is indigenous to the Indian subcontinent and the African continent, and contains numerous phytochemicals of pharmacological importance, such as reserpine and yohimbine. The composition of phytochemicals are a bit different in the species found in Africa when compared to the species that is found in the Indian subcontinent. Reserpine was once used to lower blood pressure, but the drug had numerous side effects that led to its discontinuation. However, it can be cultivated for its scent, and to make your garden yoga exercises more pleasant.

Gotu Kola

This herb belongs to the parsley family and is indigenous to the Indian subcontinent. It balances the crown chakra, and improves the functions of the neurotransmitters that are found in the nervous system. Cognitive health is also improved with its consumption.

Lemongrass

This herb helps to hone your senses and focus, and therefore, your tendency to procrastinate decreases to a substantial degree. It has effects that are similar to camellia.

Camellia

This is a genus of flowering plants that includes about 220 species of beautiful plants. They can be cultivated to get beautiful flowers that are used to make tea. The tea contains a non-protein amino acid, called L-theanine. This compound in the tea modulates mood and induces a state of relaxed alertness, as it increases the formation of alpha waves in the brain. The tea can be consumed before a session of meditation or yoga.

Hibiscus

This flowering plant can be grown in your garden to make tea out of the flowers. The anthocyanins present in the flowers lend a beautiful color to the tea. Hibiscus tea has an effect that is similar to that of chamomile and camellia, as it calms the senses and relieves anxiety. A cup of tea before your yoga session can improve your sense of calm.

Danshen

This herb is used in Chinese herbal medicine to treat atherosclerosis. It is also used to dampen feelings of aggression and mellow anger. It is particularly popular in Chinese folklore as well. Research on the mental health benefits of this herb has not been done to a considerable degree till now.

Chapter 11
The Ethics of Herbalism

The world has seen tremendous changes over the past few decades, and has become more prone to the devastating effects of the industrial revolution. Harmful industrial effluents poisoning the terrain and plumes of smoke going into the sky from industries have made humans realise that the breakthroughs of the past 150 years have come at the cost of the environment. The burgeoning human population and expansive deforestation and cattle farming have increased the greenhouse effect of these harmful gases. The enormous number of cattle that have been bred release methane from their gastrointestinal tract, which itself is a greenhouse gas and contributes to global heating. These instances of irreversible devastation have pushed mankind to adopt measures to slow the progression of the climate crisis, if it cannot be stopped completely.

Understanding Ethical Herbalism

The devastating effect of global heating and climate crisis have coerced humans to ponder over the impact that we have on the planet. Sustainable practices have become normalised that tend to subside the carbon footprint that we create on the planet. Dependence on non-biodegradable, single-use plastic has polluted the oceans, and ocean cleanup projects have been initiated that aim to mop up the debris that has been choking marine life. Fracking for crude oil has augmented the desolation of the environment, and the oil that spills from ships that sometimes capsize completely destroy the life in the vicinity of the spill. These factors have called for practices that make herbalism common among the masses but not at the expense of the environment.

Cloth bags have become normalised due to their ability to be reused. The bags have also been made by some fashion brands, so that those of us who like to go on a shopping spree in style can find them handy. The bags are made of cloth, which does absolutely no damage to the environment. Compostable bags have also been made by some companies that can be degraded by the soil when disposed of properly. The cassava root has been used by a startup in Indonesia in 2014 to make bags that are durable and biodegradable. The root lends tensile strength to the bag, but the bag can be dissolved in water, hence creating no devastating impact on the environment.

Biomaterials have been synthesised by biotechnology research companies that can be used by the fashion and textile industry. Polybion is one such company that has produced a biomaterial called Celium®, which is cellulose synthesised by bacteria cultured in fermenters. This biomaterial serves as an alternative to leather, and could help to reduce or completely eradicate reliance on actual leather that is sourced from crocodiles and perpetuates the inhumane killing methods of these reptiles by cervical dislocation. Celium® has recently been used by the Danish clothing company Ganni to make trendy jackets.

These advances in modern biotechnology have made it possible to rethink our way of living. When you go to the nursery to buy seeds, think about using reusable cloth bags instead of plastic bags. The plastic bags are made from polyethylene (polythene) that takes about 500 years to completely degrade by the environment.

Wildcrafting and Other Sustainable Sourcing practices

Although growing your own herbs is the scope of this book and lies at the epicentre of the subject-matter, this chapter also discusses how you can forage food in the wild. This practice is called wildcrafting, and deals with harvesting plants from their natural (wild) habitat. The purpose can be foraging, such as picking berries, or to look for plants for that have useful medicinal properties. Wildcrafting can be done if your house is located in an area that has lush vegetation, such as an estate located on a hilltop. You can go for wildcrafting if you have run out of your herbal stock, and the herbs that you have growing in your garden have not yet completed their growth.

Wildcrafting is an adventurous journey into the woods that strengthens your connection with nature. The activity of picking berries and looking for plants of medicinal importance requires you to be aware of the appearance of these plants. Numerous archives and book are available in public libraries that can give you an insight into this aspect of botany. Going into the woods and breathing the fresh air lightens your heart and takes away your worries, because the connection with nature is powerful and rejuvenates the mind, body, and spirit. It can be considered a holistic journey into your inner self.

Prior to venturing into the woods for foraging and wildcrafting, you need to check your municipality's website or other sources to see if this activity is legal. There are certain tracts of forests that are protected by laws, which have been enacted because forests are dwindling. The same kind of laws have also been enacted to protect oceans, and such region of the sea that make shoreline have been called Marine Protected Areas (MPAs). The Marine Protected Areas are found in the Unites States, South Africa, and some other countries. As a result of these laws, you cannot just simply deracinate a herb from a forest that is protected.

Rangers and surveillance cameras keep a watchful eye on everyone's activities, and should not do wildcrafting in such areas. Nevertheless, if the woods in the vicinity of your house do not lie in protected areas, you can forage or look for medicinal herbs. Still, beware the cunning and stealth of animals, such as mountain lions, and never venture into a forest without a licensed firearm.

Additionally, express your gratitude for anything that you find in the wild. even if you have been able to pick berries that do not come with a price tag, this is Earth's bounty that you are going to consume, and you should give thanks for whatever you find in the woods. Also, you need to be able to harvest in a way that does not impact the ecosystem. Harvest only those plants that you see in abundance, so that the population can replenish and grow again to reach healthy numbers. Also, you need to know about the life cycle of the plant, so that you can harvest the plant in way that allows it grow shoots once more. Always harvest the plants that are in abundant numbers, and leave enough plants for future foragers. It is better to go for the invasive species first. Invasive species are those that do not form a natural part of the area's ecosystem, and have been introduced as a result of the Europeans colonising the America's upon discovery of the New World. These species have been naturalised as a result of ships bringing people form the Old World.

Cultural Respect and Avoiding Appropriation

Cultural appropriation is the unacknowledged adoption of the aspects of a culture by members of another culture. This phenomenon happens in herbalism as well if you adopt a particular ritual of another culture and pass it off as something that you did all by yourself. It is a good practice to look for the rituals that are practiced in other cultures, and to incorporate them in your life. Also, spread the word about these practices and how the culture shaped the ritual through the passage of time.

Telling your family and friends about how you have been positively influenced by a ritual that is a part of another culture helps to spread positivity about that particular culture. This helps the members of that culture to be respected by other people as well. Other people might also try to adopt the ritual in an attempt to reap benefits from that practice. Cultural appropriation negatively impacts countless people who, either on purpose or inadvertently, try to pass a ritual as something that they did all by themselves. It is something that is demeaning and must be condemned, so you should consider guiding others that you see engaged in this practice about the damage that this can do to a culture.

Chapter 12

The Global Herbal Movement

There has been undeniable resurgence of herbalism that has been guided by the successful incorporation of traditional knowledge and modern science under the guise of holistic practices. This has helped breathe life into the art of traditional herbal medicine that was slowly dying out and entering a state of oblivion. Thankfully, these herbal practices have been gracefully accepted by the public, and even revered to an extent that people now actively engage in practices that can steer them away from the excessive use of medications. This has positively impacted the cultures that have given birth to this traditional knowledge, so to speak.

Herbalism in the Modern World

You would see many a people engaging in active dissemination of knowledge on social media as well, and many businesses successfully source herbs and market them in order to increase awareness pertinent to the indelible mark that traditional knowledge has embossed on the development of humanity. Contemporary times have seen an unprecedented uptick in the use of herbs, and traditional knowledge is being used in conjunction with modern medicine to make people's lives better.

Bridging Tradition and Innovation

The doctors of today and other healthcare professionals are actively engaged in the spread of traditional knowledge that sits well with modern medicine. You would even see some doctors spreading awareness about the use of natural herbs and how they can be integrated with your prescription regimen to form a holistic approach to curing your ailments. However, you should always check with your doctor before combining traditional knowledge with the use of prescription drugs. Some herbs and drugs can have interactions that can negatively impact your health. Some interactions simply reduce the absorption of one of the drugs, while other interactions can have a lethal impact on your overall well-being. So, always seek consultation of your doctor before combining herbal medicine with modern medicine.

Dr. Josh Axe is highly famous for his integrative health approach and speaks actively about the benefits of ancient practices. He is dedicated to the use of herbs and instigates people to incorporate them with their lifestyle in order to achieve a better health tier.

Cross-Cultural Exchange of Herbal Knowledge

Herbalism is a global phenomenon and each culture has its own method of concocting remedies to treat an ailment and cure a disease. Cross-cultural exchange is something that has been happening since humanity was born. Empires and kingdoms have undergone changes in their borders as a result of wars and ensuing territorial expansion. When cultures collided under the hood of a newly formed empire, new cultural interactions took place, and this morphed the way ethnicities developed. In many instances, new ethnicities were born, and the interactions between these ethnicities allowed new languages to be developed. There have been many conquering ethnicities that used to dominate a particular region and developed a lingua franca, a language that bridges different ethnicities by combining the elements of the original languages. The phenomenon of the lingua franca took place all across the globe, and these languages are dominant to this day in their respective regions.

The lingua franca is made in a way that it takes the script of one language, resembles the phonetics of another language, and has loanwords from all languages that serve as its building blocks. The lingua franca helped the conquering power establish dominance by stealthily imbuing its language into the people, because the people got to learn the language of the conquering power through the guise of developing a bridge between the ethnicities that lived under the umbrella of the massive empire. There are many examples of lingua franca in the world, including Afrikaans that is spoken in South Africa, and Urdu that is spoken in the Indian subcontinent. Afrikaans was developed using the different languages spoken by regional ethnicities in Southern Africa, including Xhosa and Zulu. These were combined with the languages of the colonial powers that had remained dominant in the region, i.e., English, German, and Dutch. Urdu was created by the Turks that ruled the Indian subcontinent in the 1000s, who amalgamated Turkish, Arabic, Farsi, and Hindi to give life to this new lingua franca. Urdu is one of the most dominant languages in the world to this day, spoken and understood by billions of people.

Herbal knowledge has undergone the same transformation through the centuries. Healers from different ethnicities used to come together to share their knowledge and learn from the experiences and regional knowledge that other healers had to offer. This made traditional knowledge in a specific region undergo changes that are hitherto unknown. We cannot really determine the extent to which Chinese medicine was influenced by the ethnicities that came under the empires that the Chinese ruled for centuries. Without any doubt, knowledge was shared by different healers from different regions, so much so that the regional records must have undergone change. However, there is no record of how exactly these events transpired. We know from global history that the breakthroughs made by a civilisation or kingdom were revered and highly sought-after by other kingdoms. This allowed other ethnicities to follow suit and refine the original idea in order to improve it and gain an evolutionary advantage over the enemy.,

Gunpowder was invented by the Chinese around the 10th and 12th centuries, but its use was refined by the Arabs who used barrels made out of bamboo and iron to channel the explosive power of the black powder to propel a projectile. This allowed three Islamic empires, namely, Ottoman, Safavid, and Mughal empire, to establish control over huge swathes of land and establish an unchallenged control. The use of herbs has undergone the same refinement in traditional knowledge, as herbal knowledge was transmitted among healers hailing from different regions. Chinese medicine is one of the oldest medical systems and many Chinese dynasties ruled huge swathes of land for centuries, allowing healers to learn the secrets of different cultures and affecting the remedies available in Chinese literature.

The exchange of ideas and blending of traditions has been a commonplace occurrence throughout history, and happens to this day. This exchange of ideas influences the way we think and process information. Herbal knowledge has been subject to the same cross-cultural influences, and allowed healers to refine their knowledge by absorbing the subject-matter related to the traditional knowledge of other cultures. The transformation that happens through absorption of the knowledge of other cultures is a spontaneous process, and has helped shape herbal knowledge.

Advocacy and Community in Herbalism

There are many social groups that are focused on advocating the use of herbs to treat minor ailments. Online chatter in these groups is focused on directing the interest of people toward the use of herbs in their lives. The transformational power of these herbs is not just limited to the alleviation of ailments, as they also uplift the mood, and allow the person using the herb to dive into their inner-self and explore their spiritual side. These communities encourage people to turn to herbalism and steer away from modern medicine.

The sense of belonging that a vibrant and thriving community lends to you strengthens your conviction about your lifestyle. Being surrounded by like-minded people who find you simpatico in this facet of life helps to fuel your dedication for a lifestyle that is fuelled by herbalism. Also, you and your community can help entice other people toward the use of herbs and expand the approach of herbalism to new people. Being a part of a community also helps you to learn more about how different herbs can be used in your life, form cooking to the alleviation of ailments. This bolsters the dedication that you have for this life, and gives you inner peace, while making you realise that you are not alone in an effort to eliminate the trend to rely on modern medicine.

Chapter 13

Building Your Herbal Community

Your journey toward a life marked by profuse use of herbs can be shared with others if you become a part of a vibrant community oozing with traditional knowledge that helps you to diversify your own knowledge about the use of these herbs. Sharing of knowledge and ancient practices can also help you make new friends that share the same newfound love that you have for herbalism. Embarking on this journey of herbalism might present hindrances at the first glance, but discovering the upside of herbalism and finding new friends that share your passions can help you settle into this life.

The Importance of Community in Herbalism

Being a part of a community can eliminate that feeling of being alone on your journey. It is like going on a ride through a scenic landscape with a friend, instead of being alone on this ride. For obvious reasons, humans are wired to be social beings, and we enjoy everything even more when we have someone by our side to share our passion for a particular thing. This fuels your energy and drive to stick to your dedication and commitment to be an enthusiast of herbal remedies.

There are numerous networking opportunities provided by forums that serve as an indispensable scaffold for you to build a community of friends and like-minded people that keep you bound with your dedication toward herbal remedies even when your confidence and commitment for herbalism start to waver. It is true that talking to new people is a thing that some of us avoid to the maximum degree, and walking into a room full of people that are absolute strangers is not easy for everyone, but doing it can help you keep abreast with the happening in the herbal world. Staying ahead of the curve, trying new-fangled herbal remedies, and spreading the word about these remedies can imbue an incessantly good feeling about yourself.

Expansion of your knowledge base through communication with new people in your network is a vital characteristic that can drive growth and help you navigate your way in a better fashion into the herbal world. Herbal remedies have even been reported to change people's lives and you need a good network of supportive people that can help you chart a better path in life. The significance of networking cannot be ignored when you think about the way it influences college students to get referrals from their supervisors and teachers. In the same way, it helps you in a different way to stick to these herbal practices. Human have been wired to be social creatures and we need to stay in the proximity of an incessant social contact on a daily basis to keep functioning properly. Not doing so makes us fall into a chasm of loneliness wherein all dedication starts to wane its grip on your heart.

Spreading word about new ideas related to herbalism can make you stand out among others and people tend to follow you as a leader. You can become a voice that people look forward to listen to on a daily basis. Networking simply has an important on your social well-being. We need social contact to keep ourselves mentally stable, and there are numerous online chatter groups that you can join, so that you do not feel alone in this endeavour.

Participation in Sharing Circles and Study Groups

Participation in sharing circles boosts your confidence in yourself and faith in the idea that have become so close to your beliefs. As discussed before, this kind of participation in groups and networking opportunities increase your visibility and people look up to you. People start to consider you an influential voice and your expertise helps you accomplish wonders. You can read enough books on this topic to allow people to think about you in ways that are hitherto unknown, as they make an effort o get in touch with you in an attempt to learn more about herbalism.

Becoming an icon of leadership in herbalism can help you gain considerable influence in today's world that is driven by social media. You can peddle your ideas and knowledge on social media networks to make life better or people in the world. People then look up to you for everything that they need to learn and this can help you gain a lot of followers. If your content reaches enough audience, you can monetise your account to start earning good money from your social media endeavours. The feeling of accomplishment that you get when someone reaches out to you to learn more about the topic that you happen to know so much about is absolutely unparalleled.

Furthermore, you might even find a good person who has enough capital to start a business venture with you. The possibilities are endless if you have good social connections who are willing to earn good money through a partnership with you. you would be making new friends along the way and expanding the horizon for your business. Keep a good and just business model for your company that allows you to reap money while adhering to a sense of morality.

Engaging With Professional Herbalists and Leaders

Engaging with professional herbalists and leaders can provide treasures of traditional knowledge for you to be able to gain better understanding of the herbal realm. Such interactions are crucial for you to gain a deeper understanding of the herbal world. The advances if the current century have made it easier for people to gain an insight into what the experts in any field have to offer to the world. This is, in big part, with thanks to the presence of social media. You would find experts in any field who have an influential voice on any professional platform or social network. The experts on these networks pitch in their ideas and remedies in the bowl form which anyone can have a taste of what they have to offer.

In the preceding century, it used to be difficult for people to gain an understanding of what they love from the comfort of their couches. The only way to gain an understanding of the professional world was to attend conferences that were organized by leading companies in a particular field. However, now you can tap into the rich vastness of the expertise of these intellectuals on your smartphone, and from the comfort of your couch. The presence of social media makes it easy for people to tune into the conferences that are also aired live on their official social media handles. The conferences are also broadcast on other networks where virtual viewers can participate in them, either through asking questions in a chat or being able to get live video coverage.

Curiosity is a good driving force that can help you bridge the gap between your current level of knowledge and the level that you aspire to be on. Olivia Amitrano (@organic_olivia) and Dr. Nicole Apelian (@nicole_apelian) are two very famous herbalists and their Instagram handles where you can follow them. Olivia Amitrano is a clinical herbalist who spreads information about creating a diet that helps you to stay healthy. Dr. Nicole Apelian is a biologist and anthropologist, and works as an African safari guide as well, because she loves interactions with the wilderness and animals. She is a herbalist as well, and contributes to the spread of traditional knowledge.

Moreover, there are some famous doctors who work to peddle herbal information to the masses. One such doctor is Dr. Josh Axe, who has millions of followers on his Instagram handle and Facebook page. Also, he is present on X, the social media platform formerly known as Twitter, and spreads herbal knowledge there as well. These famous social media personalities and many others have made it possible for herbal knowledge to be easily accessible for millions of people. Their work has served as a crucial pedestal for the field to progress in the contemporary times.

Chapter 14
The Herbalist's Toolkit

Your journey into the world of herbalism requires you to have certain tools and resources at your disposal that would be needed to learn the art of traditional knowledge. Learning is a lifelong process and you would need to have a few must-to-have books, journals, and databases that are crucial for you to learn the secrets of planting and successfully harvesting each herb. The herbs come from different species. To plan them and grow them requires you to have adequate knowledge, so that the task of growing these herbs from scratch becomes easier for you.

Essential Tools for the Herbalist

There are certain tools that are needed for you to be able to do your tasks of planting and harvesting these herbs with relative ease. Tending to these delicate plants must be done with adequate care.

A wide variety of solvents are needed for different kinds of herbal preparations. Extracts, tinctures, infusions, and poultices require you to have a range of different strengths of alcoholic beverages. Gin, vodka, tequila, and other beverages must be present in your home, so you can use them to make your herbal preparations. Essential oils and carrier oils are a must-have as well, as these are required for you to be able to effectively craft herbal preparations. Also, vinegar, such as apple cider vinegar is needed for certain herbal preparations. Honey is used to make some herbal syrups and glycerin is added to some concoctions as well. So, you need to have these items at home.

Waxes and butters are also needed if you want to make body butters and other creams. Beeswax and carnauba wax are commonly used as bases for these creams. Beeswax is extracted from honeycombs and carnauba wax comes from the carnauba palm trees that grow in Brazil. Carnauba wax is suitable if you are a vegan, because beeswax is animal-sourced wax. Butters, like cocoa butter and shea butter, are also used for making creams. These butters are added in creams and lotions by almost all cosmetic companies, as everyone loves their fragrant odor.

A kitchen-scale would come in handy when you have to make meticulous calculations and decide to weight the herbs that you have to use for your herbal preparations. Pestle and mortar are very critical elements of the whole process, as you would have to do your trituration in this receptacle with a pestle. Also, you need saucepans of various sizes and bigger pots as well if you have to make infusions, salves, and poultices.

Measuring cups and measuring spoons are some things that are already present in the kitchens of most houses. Still, if your kitchen happens to be in a dearth of these supplies, you can purchase these items from the shop. Funnels often come in handy, so try to purchase these items as well. Consider purchasing a spare coffee grinder to grind the herbs. You cannot use the one which you use to make coffee, as the odor of coffee will diminish the natural scent of the herbal preparation.

Shears are required to prune bigger plants of the plant, and you can purchase these from the nearby nursery, or from other stores. Scissors and gardening gloves are needed to perform the tasks of sowing and harvesting. You could be allergic to some of the plant material, so never come into close contact with these things. Foraging bags are essential to pack your harvest, and some very beautiful bags made out of jute are also available in the market that you can purchase for yourself.

Building Your Herbal Reference Library With Digital Resources

The global access provided by the availability of the internet has made the task of collecting literature on the herbs very easy. You can gain access into many peer-reviewed, open-access journals with a high impact factor to heighten your knowledge about the sowing, harvesting, and advantages of herbs. Journals with a high factor have publications that have a high number of citations. This means that these articles show good research that has been conducted on the concerned topic. Books are available in e-book format and you can download them from reputable online stores. These include Amazon kindle, among others. Other book banks, such as Thrift Books, Bookshop.org, and Barnes and Noble have numerous books that are available in hardcover, paperback, and e-book formats.

if you are a bit old-fashioned, you can go for paperback books and hardcover books, as sifting through the pages spreads its own odor and sits well with many people who sit well with the page instead of computer screens. These books form an indispensable resource for you to be able to gain insight into the herbal remedies that you want to learn. You can binge read and avidly learn about the herbal realm.

Tracking Your Herbal Journey

It is always a good idea to keep your own journal in which you can write the art of sowing, harvesting, and tending to plants. There are some meticulous details that cold trickle out of your mind, so it is always better to keep a journal which you can use to refer back to some ways of cultivation that you might have forgotten. Also, you can go back to these methods to have them better ingrained in your mind. Reflect on these practices to allow your mind to conjure up better ideas and new ways that you can use to cultivate and grow your herbs. Yu can also think of adding new ingredients to the herbal concoctions that you read about in order to create your own taste for the product.

You can keep recipes that you read about in different resources in your journal, so you have a better record of what you read. This is especially true if you find some recipe on the internet. Online magazines, like Cook's Illustrated, have great recipes and peddle new-fangled ideas, but these online articles can become inaccessible for due to a wide variety of reasons, so you must have them scribbled down in your journal to have a better and indelible record of the recipes that you love. Share these recipes with your loved ones and family to allow your own brand of herbalism to be spread to a wider audience. The world can be a better place if we take one small step at a time. Bundled together, these steps can have a huge impact on coming generations.

Conclusion

Herbalism has ancient roots in our planets that are intertwined with our own existence. The body heals with the application of herbal potions and poultices because our bodies are composed of the same stardust that constitutes the planet. Modern medicine has advanced to its heights through studies about plant genetics and the biochemistry and using the discovered molecular structures as templates to synthesise the same molecules in the lab. Modern research has even made derivatives of the actual molecules with enhanced pharmacophores and altered molecular morphology that allow these derivatives to have improved drug response at the site of action. Going back to the use of traditional knowledge and ancient methods can make our lives better since we would not be exposed to the devastating side effects that come with modern allopathic medicine. The variety of phytochemicals present in the plants have the potential to considerably alleviate and suppress common ailments, and their regular use bolsters your organ systems.

Cultivating your own herbal garden adds the factor of creativity and the revelry associated with growing your own herbs. Wildcrafting and foraging serve as alternatives that can be sought when your own supply still has not approached the stage of harvest. A range of infusions, salves, and potions can be made at home using many readily available ingredients in the market and at your own home. Ethical herbalism has gained sizeable traction over the years, and sustainable practices that keep the world's ecosystems in good running shape have been encouraged. The importance of communities cannot be overlooked when dedicating yourself to this life of ethical herbalism. A vibrant communities can help you feel right at home with like-minded people.

To adhere to ancient traditional knowledge is akin to strengthening your relation with Mother Earth. Therefore, the use of herbs can reconnect and reinforce these severed ties with nature.

Glossary

- **Annual Plants**: The plants that have a life cycle of one growing season., and can be harvested relatively easily without having to worry about inflicting damage to the plant. However, the plant must still be allowed to die off by natural frost rather than forcefully deracinating it out of the soil.
- **Bioaccumulation**: The process by which exogenous metals accumulate in the body and cause poisoning.
- **Bioavailability**: This is the rate and extent to which a drug becomes available at the site of action.
- **Biodegradable**: A substance that is destroyed to shreds by the forces of nature, i.e., the action of bacteria, and eventually becomes a part of the earth.
- **Biotransformation**: This is a metabolic process that happens mainly in the liver and through which water-soluble metabolites of drugs and endogenous substances are formed that can be excreted from the body.
- **Extract**: An extract has the constituents of the plant material dissolved in a solvent. Extracts have concentrated phytochemicals and can be made even

stronger by using bulkier plant material, in which case the extract is called a tincture.

• **Infusion**: These concoctions are made by allowing the pulverised herbal material to be dissolved in water or some other solvent. Infusions can be of weak or strong strength.

• **Organic Synthesis**: A method of chemical synthesis based in the lab that allows molecules to be manufactured. An auxiliary of organic synthesis is called total synthesis, as the new molecule is designed from scratch.

• **Parchment**: This used to be untanned animal skin that was used a writing material. Goats, sheep, and young calves were used to make parchment that served as the medium of writing for more than two millennia.

• **Perennial Plants**: The plants that have a life cycle of more than two years and mostly form woody stems as they mature. They are harvested carefully, so that the stem does not get damaged, which needs to regrow shoots.

• **pH**: This is called the power of the hydrogen. This measures the concentration of hydrogen ions in a solution. The greater the hydrogen ions, the more acidic the solution, and the lower the pH.

• **Pharmacognosy**: An interdisciplinary field at the crossroads between botany and pharmacology, which has burgeoned into an area of scientific knowledge that details the composition of medicinal plants and the extraction of phytochemicals.

• **Phylogeography**: The historical scenarios that shape the geographic distribution of various genealogical lineages of plants and animals.

• **Prostaglandins**: These are hormone-like substances that are produces by some organs (brain, lungs, kidneys) and are present in some body fluids, including that in the uterus and semen. They cause the contraction of smooth muscles, such as those in the uterus, and induce labor. Also, they act as mediators in the process of inflammation and produce mucus in the stomach. NSAIDs have a mechanism of actions that allows the drugs to block the production of prostaglandins, thereby predisposing the stomach wall to peptic ulceration. There are nine classes of prostaglandins (e.g., PGA-I). Synthetic prostaglandins, like dinoprostone, is used to induce labor and case abortion. Others include misoprostol and latanoprost that are used to treat peptic ulcers and glaucoma respectively.

References

Adelmann, M. (2013, May 6). How To Make Herb-Infused Oils. Herbal Academy. https://theherbalacademy.com/herb-infused-oils/

Beaulieu, D. (2023, March 29). Learn Everything You Need to Know to Start a Garden From Scratch. The Spruce. https://www.thespruce.com/how-to-start-a-garden-from-scratch-2132778

Cohn, R. (2013, May 1). The Life Story of The Oldest Tree on Earth. Yale Environment360. https://e360.yale.edu/features/peter_crane_history_of_ginkgo_earths_oldest_tree

Deering, S. (2019, February 28). Nature's 9 Most Powerful Medicinal Plants and the Science Behind Them. Healthline. https://www.healthline.com/health/most-powerful-medicinal-plants

Evans, W. C. (2009). Pharmacognosy (16th ed.). Elsevier Saunders. (Original work published 1934)

Gillette, B. (2022, October 4). How to Harvest Herbs ad Keep Them Growing. The Spruce. https://www.thespruce.com/harvesting-herbs-for-growth-5270569

Jeanroy, A. (2022, April 1). Learn How to Make the Perfect Herbal Infusion at Home. The Spruce Eats. https://

www.thespruceeats.com/how-to-make-an-herbal-infusion-1762142

Justis, A. (2016, October 5). How to make an herbal syrup. Herbal Academy. https://theherbalacademy.com/herbal-syrup/

Lieberman, C. (2021, May 3). Basics of Foraging and Wildcrafting. Wild Abundance. https://www.wildabundance.net/blog/basics-of-foraging-and-wildcrafting/

Sams, T. (2020, August 10). Herbal Elixir Recipe for Stress Relief. Blog.mountainroseherbs.com. https://blog.mountainroseherbs.com/herbal-elixir-recipe-for-stress-relief

Did You Enjoy Your Journey With Us?

Thank you for choosing *The Lost Book of Herbal Remedies*.
We hope you enjoyed the adventure
as much as we loved bringing it to you.
If this book made you smile, think, or inspired you in any way,
we'd be delighted to hear your thoughts!

Share Your Experience!
Your feedback not only supports our work
but also helps fellow readers to discover new journeys.
Please take a moment to leave a review on Amazon.
Just scan the QR code below to share your valuable insights.
Every word you write is immensely appreciated!

Thank you once again for being a part of this wonderful community of
readers. We can't wait to hear from you!